The bronzed killer and his brothers

"Hepatomegaly

Hemochromatosis

Wilson's disease"

Acknowledgements

"Do not thank God who does not thank people" talk about the Prophet Muhammad peace be upon him, Narrated by Abu Dawood and Tirmidhi. I would like to thank my family, my mom and dad and brothers and sons Nooran , Abobker, Alaa, Lina and Abdol-Rahman and Create Space and Amazon companies and every one works on it on the mighty effort that both spend and will spend for the reach of these arts to her fans from the readers.
Dr / Osama Ahmed Bahudila

Hepatomegaly

Applied anatomy:

Normal liver structure and blood supply:
the liver shaped somewhat like a football
and is located in the upper right quadrant
of your abdomen below your diaphragm
and between your right nipple and the last
rib on your right side. The liver is usually
about 7.5 centimetres in women and 10.5
centimetres in men. It may be 3 centimetres
larger or smaller and still be normal. The
size and weight of your liver is increases
with your age and body weight. Sex and
body shape also influence the size of your
liver.

The liver weighs 1.2–1.5 kg. It is classically
divided into left and right lobes by the falciform
ligament, but a more useful functional division
is into the right and left hemilivers, based on
blood supply. These are further divided into
eight segments according to subdivisions of
the hepatic and portal veins. Each segment
has its own branch of the hepatic artery and
biliary tree. The segmental anatomy of the liver
has an important influence on imaging and
treatment of liver tumours, given the increasing
use of surgical resection. A liver segment is
made up of multiple smaller units known as
lobules, comprised of a central vein, radiating
sinusoids separated from each other by single
liver cell (hepatocyte) plates, and peripheral
portal tracts. The functional unit of the liver is
the hepatic acinus.

Blood flows into the acinus via a single branch
of the portal vein and hepatic artery situated
centrally in the portal tracts. Blood flows

outwards along the hepatic sinusoids into one of several tributaries of the hepatic vein at the periphery of the acinus. Bile, formed by active and passive excretion by hepatocytes into channels called cholangioles which lie between them, flows in the opposite direction from the periphery of the acinus.

The cholangioles converge in interlobular bile ducts in the portal tracts. The hepatocytes in each acinus lie in three zones, depending on their position relative to the portal tract. Those in zone 1 are closest to the terminal branches of the portal vein and hepatic artery, and are richly supplied with oxygenated blood, and blood containing the highest concentration of nutrients and toxins. Conversely, hepatocytes in zone 3 are furthest from the portal tracts and closest to the hepatic veins, and are therefore relatively hypoxic and exposed to lower concentrations of nutrients and toxins compared to zone 1. The different perfusion and toxin exposure patterns, and thus vulnerability, of hepatocytes in the different zones contribute to the often-patchy nature of liver injury.

Liver cells:

Hepatocytes comprise 80% of liver cells. The remaining 20% are the endothelial cells lining the sinusoids, epithelial cells lining the intrahepatic bile ducts, cells of the immune system (including macrophages (Kupffer cells) and unique populations of atypical lymphocytes),and a key population of non-parenchymal cells called stellate or Ito cells. Endothelial cells line the sinusoids, a network of capillary vessels that differ from other capillary beds in the body in that there is no basement membrane. The endothelial cells have gaps between them (fenestrae) of about 0.1 micron in diameter, allowing free flow of fluid and particulate matter to the hepatocytes. Individual hepatocytes are separated from the leaky sinusoids by the space of Disse, which contains stellate cells that store vitamin A and play an important part in regulating liver blood flow. They may also be immunologically active and play a role in the liver's contribution to defence against pathogens.

The key role of stellate cells in terms of pathology is in the development of hepatic fibrosis, the precursor of cirrhosis. They undergo activation in response to cytokines produced following liver injury, differentiating into myofibroblasts, which are the major producers of the collagen-rich matrix that forms fibrous tissue.

Blood supply:

The liver is unique as an organ as it has dual perfusion, receiving a majority of its supply via the portal vein, which drains blood from the gut via the splanchnic circulation and is the principal route for nutrient trafficking to the liver, and a minority from the hepatic artery. The portal venous contribution is 50–90%. The dual perfusion system, and the variable contribution from portal vein and hepatic artery, can have important effects on the clinical expression of liver ischaemia (which typically exhibits a less dramatic pattern than ischaemia in other organs, a fact that can sometimes lead to it being missed clinically), and can raise practical challenges in liver transplant surgery.

Biliary system and gallbladder:

Hepatocytes provide the driving force for bile flow by creating osmotic gradients of bile acids, which form micelles in bile (bile acid-dependent bile flow), and of sodium (bile acid-independent bile flow). Bile is secreted by hepatocytes and flows from cholangioles to the biliary canaliculi. The canaliculi join to form larger intrahepatic bile ducts, which in turn merge to form the right and left hepatic ducts. These ducts join as they emerge from the liver to form the common hepatic duct, which becomes the common bile duct after joining the cystic duct. The common bile duct is approximately 5 cm long and 4–6 mm wide. The distal portion of the duct passes through the head of the pancreas and usually joins the pancreatic duct before entering the duodenum through the ampullary sphincter (sphincter of Oddi). It should be noted, though, that the anatomy of the lower common bile duct can vary widely.

Common bile duct pressure is maintained by rhythmic contraction and relaxation of the sphincter of Oddi; this pressure exceeds gallbladder pressure in the fasting state, so that bile normally flows into the gallbladder, where it is concentrated tenfold by resorption of water and electrolytes.

The gallbladder is a pear-shaped sac typically lying under the right hemiliver, with its fundus located anteriorly behind the tip of the 9th costal cartilage. Anatomical variation is common and should be considered when assessing patients clinically and radiologically.

The function of the gallbladder is to concentrate, and provide a reservoir for, bile. Gallbladder tone is maintained by vagal activity, and cholecystokinin released from the duodenal mucosa during feeding causes gallbladder contraction and reduces sphincter pressure, so that bile flows into the duodenum. The body and neck of the gallbladder pass postero-medially towards the porta hepatis, and the cystic duct then joins it to the common hepatic duct. The cystic duct mucosa has prominent crescentic folds (valves of Heister), giving it a beaded appearance on cholangiography.

Hepatic function:

Your liver is a very hearty organ that is able to grow back even after large portions of it have been surgically removed. It performs many functions that are essential to your health. Liver cells produce bile, a yellowish green liquid that helps you digest fats. Your liver also stores glucose in the form of glycogen. If you do not eat enough, your liver releases glucose into your blood to keep your brain and other organs functioning.

The liver has multiple functions, including key roles in metabolism, control of infection, elimination of toxins and by-products of metabolism.

Carbohydrate, amino acid and lipid metabolism:

The liver plays a central role in carbohydrate, lipid and amino acid metabolism, and is also involved in metabolising drugs and environmental toxins. An important and increasingly recognised role for the liver is in the integration of metabolic pathways, regulating the response of the body to feeding and starvation.

Abnormality in metabolic pathways and their regulation can play an important role both in liver disease (e.g. non-alcoholic fatty liver disease (NAFLD)) and in diseases that are not conventionally regarded as diseases of the liver (such as type II diabetes mellitus and inborn errors of metabolism). Hepatocytes have specific pathways to handle each of the nutrients absorbed from the gut and carried to the liver via the portal vein. • Amino acids from dietary proteins are used for synthesis of plasma proteins, including albumin.

The liver produces 8–14 g of albumin per day, and this plays a critical role in maintaining oncotic pressure in the vascular space and in the transport of small molecules like bilirubin, hormones and drugs throughout the body.

Amino acids those are not required for the productions of new proteins are broken down, with the amino group being converted ultimately to urea.

• Following a meal, more than half of the glucose absorbed is taken up by the liver and stored as glycogen or converted to glycerol and fatty acids, thus preventing hyperglycaemia.

During fasting, glycogen is broken down to release glucose (gluconeogenesis), thereby preventing hypoglycaemia.

The liver plays a central role in lipid metabolism, producing very low-density lipoproteins and further metabolising low- and high-density lipoproteins. Dysregulation of lipid metabolism is thought to have a critical role in the pathogenesis of NAFLD. Lipids are now recognised to play a key part in the pathogenesis of hepatitis C, facilitating viral entry into hepatocytes.

Clotting factors:

The liver produces key proteins that are involved in the coagulation cascade. Many of these coagulation factors (II, VII, IX and X) are post-translationally modified by vitamin K-dependent enzymes, and their synthesis is impaired in vitamin K deficiency. Reduced clotting factor synthesis is an important and easily accessible biomarker of liver function in the setting of liver injury. Prothrombin time (PT; or the International Normalised Ratio, INR) is therefore one of the most important clinical tools available for the assessment of hepatocyte function. Note that the deranged PT or INR seen in liver disease may not directly equate to increased bleeding risk, as these tests do not capture the concurrent reduced synthesis of *anticoagulant* factors, including protein C and protein S. In general, therefore, correction of PT using blood products before minor invasive procedures should be guided by clinical risk rather than the absolute value of the PT.

Bilirubin metabolism and bile:

The liver plays a central role in the metabolism of bilirubin and is responsible for the production of bile. Between 425 and 510 mmol (250–300 mg) of unconjugated bilirubin is produced from the catabolism of haem daily. Bilirubin in the blood is normally almost all unconjugated and, because it is not water-soluble, is bound to albumin and does not pass into the urine.

Unconjugated bilirubin is taken up by hepatocytes at the sinusoidal membrane, where it is conjugated in the endoplasmic reticulum by UDP-glucuronyl transferase, producing bilirubin mono- and diglucuronide. Impaired conjugation by this enzyme is a cause of inherited hyperbilirubinaemias. These bilirubin conjugates are water-soluble and are exported into the bile canaliculi by specific carriers on the hepatocyte membranes. The conjugated bilirubin is excreted in the bile and passes into the duodenal lumen.

Once in the intestine, conjugated bilirubin is metabolised by colonic bacteria to form stercobilinogen, which may be further oxidised to stercobilin. Both stercobilinogen and stercobilin are then excreted in the stool, contributing to its brown colour. Biliary obstruction results in reduced stercobilinogen in the stool, and the stools become pale. A small amount of stercobilinogen (4 mg/day) is absorbed from the bowel, passes through the liver, and is excreted in the urine, where it is known as urobilinogen or, following further oxidisation, urobilin.

The liver secretes 1–2 L of bile daily. Bile contains bile acids (formed from cholesterol), phospholipids, bilirubin and cholesterol.

Several biliary transporter proteins have been identified. Mutations in genes encoding these proteins have been identified in inherited intrahepatic biliary diseases presenting in childhood, and in adult-onset disease such as intrahepatic cholestasis of pregnancy and gallstone formation.

Storage of vitamins and minerals:

Vitamins A, D and B12 are stored by the liver in large amounts, while others, such as vitamin K and folate, are stored in smaller amounts and disappear rapidly if dietary intake is reduced. The liver is also able to metabolise vitamins to more active compounds, e.g.7-dehydrocholesterol to 25(OH) vitamin D. Vitamin K is a fat-soluble vitamin and so the inability to absorb fat soluble vitamins, as occurs in biliary obstruction, results in a coagulopathy. The liver also stores minerals such as iron, in ferritin and haemosiderin, and copper, which is excreted in bile.

Immune regulation:

Approximately 9% of the normal liver is composed of immune cells. Cells of the innate immune system include Kupffer cells derived from blood monocytes, the liver macrophages and natural killer (NK) cells, as well as 'classical' B and T cells of the adaptive immune response. An additional type of atypical lymphocyte, with phenotypic features of both T cells and NK cells is thought to play an important role in host defence, through linking of innate and adaptive immunity. The enrichment of such cells in the liver reflects the unique importance of the liver in preventing microorganisms from the gut entering the systemic circulation. Kupffer cells constitute the largest single mass of tissue-resident macrophages in the body and account for 80% of the phagocytic capacity of this system. They remove aged and damaged red blood cells, bacteria, viruses, antigen–antibody complexes and endotoxin.

They also produce a wide variety of inflammatory mediators that can act locally or may be released into the systemic circulation. The immunological environment of the liver is unique in that antigens presented within it tend to induce immunological tolerance. This is of importance in liver transplantation, where classical major histocompatibility (MHC) barriers may be crossed, and also in chronic viral infections, when immune responses may be attenuated.

The mechanisms that underlie this phenomenon have not been fully defined.

Definition:

Hepatomegaly is the enlargement of your liver. An enlarged liver is a sign that something is seriously wrong with your health. Hepatomegaly is always a cause for medical evaluation, although not all of the underlying conditions that cause it are medical emergencies.

Causes:

Hepatomegaly may occur as the result of a general enlargement of the liver or because of primary or secondary liver tumour (Box 1). The most common liver tumour in Western countries is liver metastasis, whereas primary liver cancer complicating chronic viral hepatitis is more common in the Far East. Unlike metastases, neuro-endocrine tumours typically cause massive hepatomegaly but without significant weight loss.

Cirrhosis can be associated with either

hepatomegaly or reduced liver size in advanced disease. Although all causes of cirrhosis can involve hepatomegaly, it is much more common in alcoholic liver disease and haemochromatosis. Hepatomegaly may resolve in patients with alcoholic cirrhosis when they stop drinking.

Box 1: **Causes of change in liver size large liver (hepatomegaly)**:

1- Liver metastases (where cancer cells have spread from other parts of the body).

2- Multiple or large hepatic cysts

3-Cirrhosis (early): NAFLD, alcohol, haemochromatosis

4-Hepatic vein outflow obstruction

5-Infiltration: amyloid

6-metastatic cancer

7- congestive heart failure

8-lymphoma

9-alcoholic hepatitis

10-fatty liver caused by total parenteral nutrition (TPN)

Some other causes of hepatomegaly are:

11-infectious hepatitis (hepatitis A, B, or C, or mononucleosis)

12-toxic hepatitis

13-obstruction of your bile ducts or gall bladder

14-Gaucher's disease (a disorder that causes fatty substances to build up in your liver)

15-hemachromatosis (a disease that causes iron to build up in your liver

16-Wilson's disease (a disease that causes copper to build up in your liver)

17-fluid-filled cysts

Small liver:

Cirrhosis (late)

Alcoholic Liver Disease :

Damage to the liver from excessive drinking can lead to ALD. Years of alcohol abuse cause the liver to become inflamed and swollen. This damage can also cause scarring known as cirrhosis.

Congestive Heart Failure (CHF):

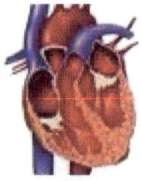 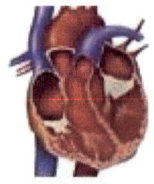

Normal   CHF

Fig 1; **Congestive Heart Failure (CHF).** Congestive heart failure is a chronic condition that affects the four chambers of the heart. Early symptoms include fatigue and weight gain. Irregular heart beat and wheezing indicate a worsening.

Cirrhosis:

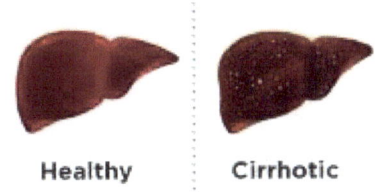

Healthy   Cirrhotic

Fig 2: **Cirrhosis.**

Image attribution:

Cirrhosis is severe scarring and poor function of the liver caused by long-term exposure to toxins such as alcohol or viral infections. Certain medications and disorder can also cause cirrhosis.

Hepatitis;

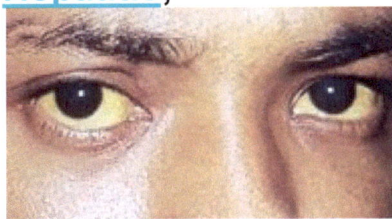

Fig3: Hepatitis.

Hepatitis is swelling and inflammation of the liver. It's usually caused by a viral infection. There are several types of hepatitis, including: A, B, C, D, and E.

Symptoms may not occur until liver damage occurs.

Liver Cancer:

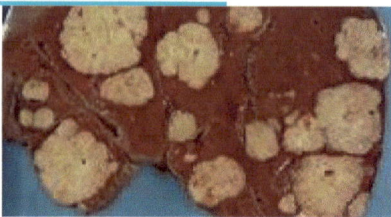

Fig 4: **Liver Cancer.**

Liver cancer causes destruction of liver cells and interferes with the ability of the liver to function normally. Cancer that originates in the liver can spread from the liver to other parts of the body.

Hyperlipidemia:

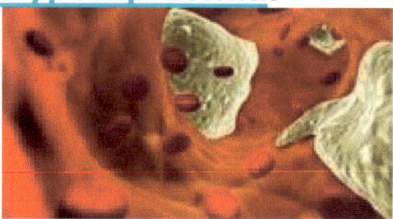

Fig 5: **Hyperlipidemia.**

Cholesterol is a natural substance, but too much of it can clog blood vessels and lead to heart attack or stroke. High cholesterol levels can also cause yellow deposits in the eyes or in tendons.

Chronic Lymphocytic Leukaemia:

Leukaemia is a type of cancer that affects the blood and blood-forming tissues. There are many types of leukaemia, each affecting different kinds of blood cells.

Hepatic Vein Thrombosis (Budd-Chiari Syndrome):

Hepatic vein thrombosis (HVT) is an obstruction in the veins of the liver caused by a blood clot. This condition blocks blood flow from the liver to the heart.

Familial Combined Hyperlipidemia

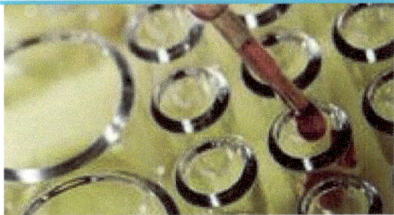

Fig6

Familial combined hyperlipidemia is an inherited disorder that causes high cholesterol and high levels of triglycerides. Some individuals have no physical symptoms from the disease. For others, it may cause chest pain.

Hyperlipoproteinemia_Type_IV:

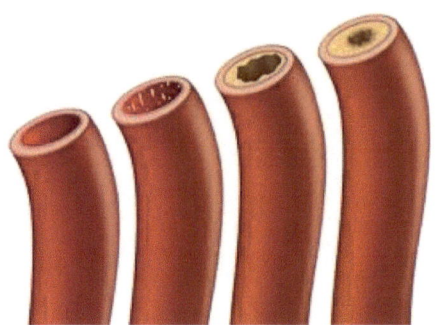

Fig 7

Hyperlipoproteinemia type IV leads to higher-than-normal triglyceride level due to a genetic defect. This may cause atherosclerosis and increase risk for certain heart conditions, including coronary artery disease.

Gaucher's_Disease:

Gaucher disease is an inherited condition in which your body does not store fatty materials (called lipids) correctly. Fatty substances can build up around your vital organs, including your liver, spleen, lungs, and bones.

Metabolic Syndrome X :

Metabolic syndrome X is a group of five

risk factors that can increase your chance of developing cardiovascular diseases, such as heart disease, diabetes, and stroke. The risk factors include: increased blood pressure...

Pericarditis:

Pericarditis is the inflammation of the sac that surrounds your heart. The sac is a double-layered membrane called the pericardium. The pericardium protects your heart and helps it function properly.

Adult-Onset Still's Disease:

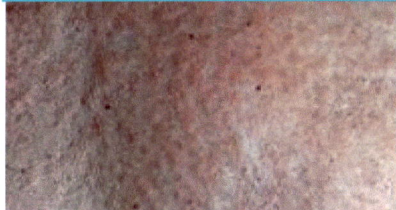

Fig 8 .

This relatively rare inflammatory condition begins with fever and may lead to arthritis. Women and people between the ages of 16 and 46 are most at risk.

Hyperlipoproteinemia:

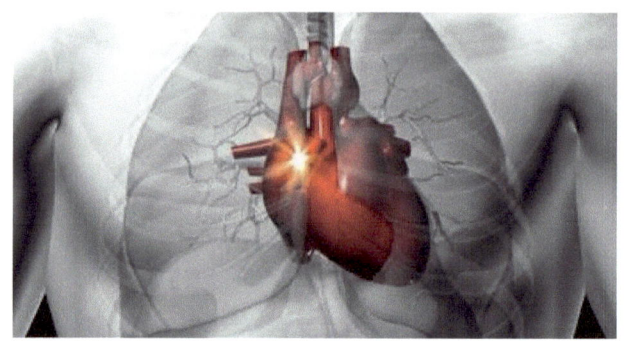

Fig 9.

Hyperlipoproteinemia is a common disorder that results in high levels of lipids circulating in the blood. This can cause pancreatitis, abdominal pain, enlarged liver and other symptoms.

Diagnosis:

To find out why you have hepatomegaly, your doctor may order a variety of tests, such as:

CBC (complete blood count to evaluate general health).

Liver enzymes.

Abdominal X-ray (non-invasive X-ray study that serves as a quick, initial evaluation of abdominal organs).

- CAT scan of the abdomen (X-rays obtain high resolution images of the liver and other abdominal organs to evaluate liver size.) (Wolf, 1990).
- MRI of the abdomen (magnetic resonance to make high resolution images of the abdominal organs).
- Ultrasound of the abdomen (sound waves to evaluate the liver and other abdominal organs).
- Liver biopsy (an invasive test that takes a small sample of liver for microscopic examination to make a diagnosis).

Investigations play an important role in the management of liver disease in three settings:
• Identification of the presence of liver disease.
• establishing the aetiology.
• understanding disease severity (in particular, identification of cirrhosis with its complications).
When planning investigations it is important to be clear as to which of these goals is being addressed.
Suspicion of the presence of liver disease is normally based on blood biochemistry abnormality ('liver function tests', or 'LFTs'),

undertaken either as a result of clinical suspicion or, increasingly, in the setting of health screening. Less commonly, suspicion arises after a structural abnormality is identified on imaging.

Aetiology is typically established through a combination of history, specific blood tests and, where appropriate, imaging and liver biopsy.

Staging of disease (in essence, the identification of cirrhosis) is largely histological, although there is increasing interest in non-invasive approaches, including novel imaging modalities, serum markers of fibrosis and the use of predictive scoring systems.

The aims of investigation in patients with suspected liver disease are shown in Box 2.

Box 2: Aims of investigations in patients with suspected liver disease

• **Detect hepatic abnormality**
• **Measure the severity of liver damage**
• **Detect the pattern of liver function test abnormality: hepatitic
or obstructive/cholestatic**
• **Identify the specific cause**
• **Investigate possible complications**

Liver blood biochemistry:

Liver blood biochemistry (LFTs) includes the measurement of serum bilirubin, aminotransferases, alkaline phosphatase, gamma-glutamyl transferase and albumin. Most analytes measured by LFTs are not truly 'function' tests but, given that they are released by:

• Detect hepatic abnormality.
• Measure the severity of liver damage.

• Detect the pattern of liver function test abnormality: hepatitis or obstructive/cholestatic
• Identify the specific cause.
• Investigate possible complications injured hepatocytes; instead provide biochemical evidence of liver cell damage. Liver function per se is best assessed by the serum albumin, PT and bilirubin because of the role played by the liver in synthesis of albumin and clotting factors and in clearance of bilirubin.

Although LFT abnormalities are often non-specific, the patterns are frequently helpful in directing further investigations. Also, levels of bilirubin and albumin and the PT are related to clinical outcome in patients with severe liver disease, reflected by their use in several prognostic scores: the Child–Pugh and MELD scores in cirrhosis, the Glasgow score in alcoholic hepatitis and the King's College Hospital criteria for liver transplantation in acute liver failure.

Bilirubin and albumin:

The degree of elevation of bilirubin can reflect the degree of liver damage. A raised bilirubin often occurs earlier in the natural history of biliary disease (e.g. primary biliary cirrhosis) than in disease of the liver parenchyma (e.g. cirrhosis) where the hepatocytes are primarily involved. Swelling of the liver within its capsule in inflammation can, however, sometimes impair bile flow and cause an elevation of bilirubin level that is disproportionate to the degree of liver injury. Caution is therefore needed in interpreting the level of liver injury purely on the basis of bilirubin elevation.

Serum albumin levels are often low in patients with liver disease. This is due to a change in the volume of distribution of albumin, and reduced synthesis. Since the plasma half-life of albumin is about 2 weeks, albumin levels may be normal in acute liver failure but are almost always reduced in chronic liver failure.

Alanine aminotransferase and aspartate aminotransferase:

Alanine aminotransferase (ALT) and aspartate aminotransferase (AST) are located in the cytoplasm of the hepatocyte; AST is also located in the hepatocyte mitochondria. Although both transaminase enzymes are widely distributed, expression of ALT outside the liver is relatively low and this enzyme is therefore considered more specific for hepatocellular damage.

Large increases of aminotransferase activity favour hepatocellular damage, and this pattern of LFT abnormality is known as 'hepatitic'.

Alkaline phosphatase and gamma-glutamyl transferase alkaline phosphatase (ALP) is the collective name given to several different enzymes that hydrolyse phosphate esters at alkaline pH. These enzymes are widely distributed in the body, but the main sites of production are the liver, gastrointestinal tract, bone, placenta and kidney. ALPs are post-translationally modified, resulting in the production of several different isoenzymes, which differ in abundance in different tissues. ALP enzymes in the liver are located in cell membranes of the hepatic sinusoids and the biliary canaliculi. Accordingly, levels rise with intrahepatic and extrahepatic biliary obstruction and with sinusoidal obstruction, as occurs in infiltrative liver disease.

Pattern	AST/ALT	GGT	ALP
Box 3 'Hepatitic 'and' cholestatic'/'obstructive' Liver function tests.			
Biliary obstruction	↑	↑↑	↑↑↑
Hepatitis	↑↑↑	↑	↑
Alcohol/enzyme-inducing Drugs	N/↑	↑↑	N

N = normal; ↑ mild elevation (< twice normal); ↑↑ moderate elevation
(2–5 times normal); ↑↑↑ marked elevation (> 5 times normal).
(ALT = alanine aminotransferase; ALP = alkaline phosphatase; AST = aspartate aminotransferase; GGT = gamma-glutamyltransferase)

Box 4: **Drugs that increase levels of gamma-glutamyltransferase**
•Barbiturates
• Carbamazepine
• Ethanol
• Griseofulvin
• Isoniazid
• Rifampicin
• Phenytoin

Gamma-glutamyl transferase (GGT) is a microsomal enzyme found in many cells and tissues of the body.
The highest concentrations are located in the liver, where it is produced by hepatocytes and by the epithelium lining small bile ducts. The function of GGT is to transfer glutamyl groups from gamma-glutamyl peptides to other peptides and amino acids.

The pattern of a modest increase in aminotransferase activity and large increases in ALP and GGT activity favours biliary obstruction and is commonly described as 'cholestatic' or 'obstructive' (Box 3). Isolated elevation of the serum GGT is relatively common, and may occur during ingestion of microsomal enzyme-inducing drugs, including alcohol (Box 4), but also in NAFLD.

Other biochemical tests:

Other widely available biochemical tests may become altered in patients with liver disease:

• Hyponatraemia occurs in severe liver disease due to increased production of antidiuretic hormone.

• Serum urea may be reduced in hepatic failure, whereas levels of urea may be increased following gastrointestinal haemorrhage.

• When high levels of urea are accompanied by raised bilirubin, high serum creatinine and low urinary sodium, this suggests hepatorenal failure, which carries a grave prognosis.

• Significantly elevated ferritin suggests haemochromatosis. Modest elevations can be seen in inflammatory disease and alcohol excess.

Haematological tests:

Blood count:

The peripheral blood count is often abnormal and can give a clue to the underlying diagnosis:

• *A normochromic normocytic anaemia* may reflect recent gastrointestinal haemorrhage, whereas chronic blood loss is characterised by a hypochromic microcytic anaemia secondary to iron deficiency. A high erythrocyte mean cell volume (macrocytosis) is associated with alcohol misuse, but target cells in any jaundiced patient also result in a macrocytosis. Macrocytosis can persist for a long period of time after alcohol cessation, making it a poor marker of ongoing consumption.

• *Leucopenia* may complicate portal hypertension and hypersplenism, whereas leucocytosis may occur with cholangitis, alcoholic hepatitis and hepatic abscesses. Atypical lymphocytes are seen in infectious mononucleosis, which may be complicated by an acute hepatitis.

• *Thrombocytopenia* is common in cirrhosis and is due to reduced platelet production, and increased breakdown because of hypersplenism.

Thrombopoietin, required for platelet production, is produced in the liver and levels fall with worsening liver function. Thus platelet levels are usually more depressed than white cells and haemoglobin in the presence of hypersplenismin patients with cirrhosis. A low platelet countis often an indicator of chronic liver disease, particularly in the context of hepatomegaly.

Thrombocytosis is unusual in patients with liver disease but may occur in those with active gastrointestinal haemorrhage and, rarely, in hepatocellular carcinoma.

Coagulation tests:

These are often abnormal in patients with liver disease.

The normal half-lives of the vitamin K-dependent coagulation factors in the blood are short (5–72 hours) and so changes in the prothrombin time occur relatively quickly following liver damage; these changes provide valuable prognostic information in patients with both acute and chronic liver failure. An increased PT is evidence of severe liver damage in chronic liver disease. Vitamin K does not reverse this deficiency if it is due to liver disease, but will correct the PT if the cause is vitamin K deficiency, as may occur with biliary obstruction due to non-absorption of fat-soluble vitamins.

Immunological tests:

A variety of tests are available to evaluate the aetiology of hepatic disease (Boxes 5 and 6). The presence of liver-related autoantibodies can be suggestive of the presence of autoimmune liver disease (although false positive results can occur in non-autoimmune inflammatory disease such as NAFLD). Elevation in overall
• Hepatitis B surface antigen
• Hepatitis C antibody

Boxes 5: Chronic liver disease screen
• **Hepatitis B surface antigen** • **Hepatitis C antibody** • **Liver autoantibodies** **(antinuclear antibody,** **smooth muscle antibody,** **antimitochondrial antibody)** • **Immunoglobulins** • **Ferritin** • **α1-antitrypsin** • **Caeruloplasmin**

Boxes 6 : How to identify the cause of LFT abnormality:

Diagnosis	Clinical clue	Initial test	Additional tests
Alcoholic liver disease	History	LFTs AST > ALT; high MCV	Random blood alcohol
Non-alcoholic fatty liver disease (NAFLD)	Metabolic syndrome (central obesity, diabetes, hypertension)	LFTs	Liver biopsy
Chronic hepatitis B	Injection drug use; blood transfusion	HBsAg	HBeAg, HBeAb HBV-DNA
Chronic hepatitis C		HCV antibody	HCV-RNA
Primary biliary cirrhosis	Itching; raised ALP	AMA	Liver biopsy
Primary sclerosing cholangitis	Inflammatory bowel Disease	MRCP	ANCA
Autoimmune hepatitis	Other autoimmune diseases	ASMA, ANA, LKM, immunoglobulin	Liver biopsy
Haemochromatosis	Diabetes /joint pain	Transferrin saturation, ferritin	HFE gene test
Wilson's disease	Neurological signs; haemolysis	Caeruloplasmin	24-hr urinary copper
α_1-antitrypsin	Lung disease	α_1-antitrypsin level	α_1-antitrypsin genotype
Drug-induced liver disease	Drug/herbal remedy history	LFTs	Liver biopsy
Coeliac disease	Malabsorption	Endomysial antibody	Small bowel biopsy

ALP = alkaline phosphatase; ALT = alanine aminotransferase; AMA = antimitochondrial antibody; ANA = antinuclear antibody; ANCA = antineutrophil cytoplasmic antibodies; ASMA = anti-smooth muscle antibody; AST =

• Liver autoantibodies (antinuclear antibody, smooth muscle antibody, antimitochondrial antibody)
• Immunoglobulins
• Ferritin
• α1-antitrypsin
• Caeruloplasmin

Serum immunoglobulin levels can also be suggestive of autoimmunity (immunoglobulin (Ig) G and IgM).

Elevated serum IgA can be seen, often in more advanced alcoholic liver disease and NAFLD, although the association is not specific.

Imaging:

Several imaging techniques can be used to determine the site and general nature of structural lesions in the liver and biliary tree. In general, however, imaging techniques are unable to identify hepatic inflammation and have poor sensitivity for liver fibrosis unless advanced cirrhosis with portal hypertension is present.

Ultrasound:

Ultrasound is non-invasive and most commonly used as a 'first-line' test to identify gallstones, biliary obstruction (Fig. 10) or thrombosis in the hepatic vasculature. Ultrasound is good for the identification of splenomegaly and abnormalities in liver texture, but is less effective at identifying diffuse parenchymal disease.

Focal lesions, such as tumours, may not be detected if they are below 2 cm in diameter and have echogenic characteristics similar to normal liver tissue. Bubble based contrast media are now routinely used and can enhance discriminant capability. Doppler ultrasound allows blood flow in the hepatic artery, portal vein and hepatic veins to be investigated. Endoscopic ultrasound provides high-resolution images of the pancreas, biliary tree and liver.

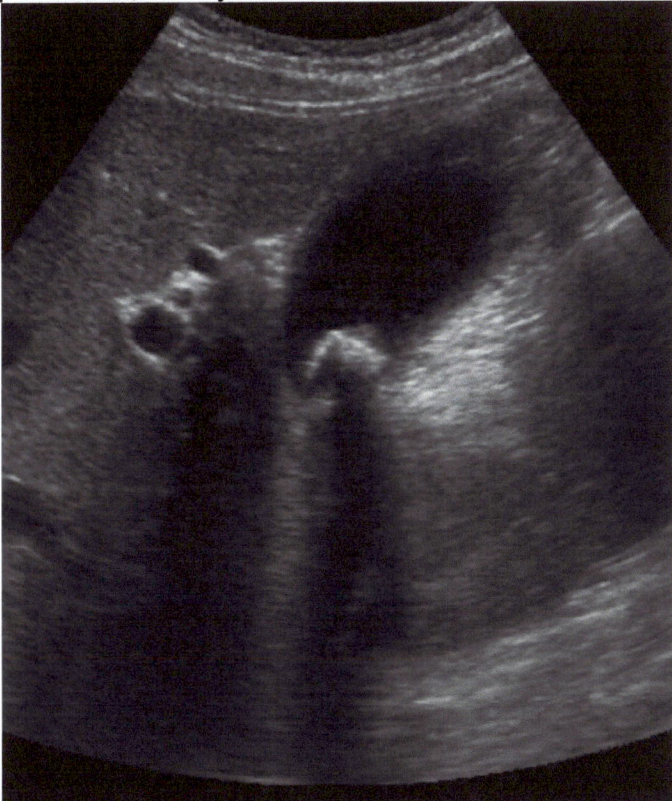

Fig. 10: Ultrasound showing a stone in the gallbladder. Stone (arrow) with acoustic shadow (S).

Computed tomography (CT) detects smaller focal lesions in the liver, especially when combined with contrast injection (Fig. 11). Magnetic resonance imaging (MRI) can also be used to localise and confirm the aetiology of focal liver lesions, particularly primary and secondary tumours.

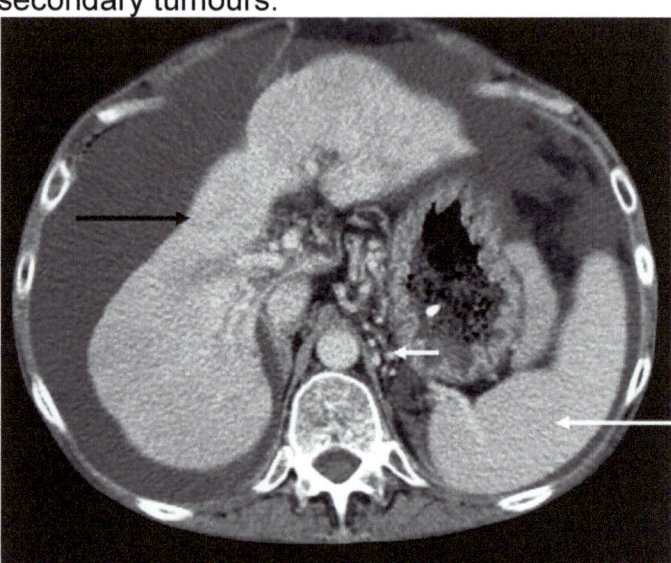

Fig. 11: CT scan in a patient with cirrhosis. The liver is small and has an irregular outline (black arrow), the spleen is enlarged (long white arrow), fluid (ascites) is seen around the liver, and collateral vessels are present around the proximal stomach (short white arrow). Hepatic angiography is seldom used nowadays as a diagnostic tool, since CT and MRI are both able to provide images of hepatic vasculature, but it still has a therapeutic role in the embolisation of vascular tumours such as

hepatocellular carcinoma. Hepatic venography is now rarely performed.

Cholangiography:

Cholangiography can be undertaken by magnetic resonance cholangiopancreatography (MRCP, Fig. 12), endoscopy (endoscopic retrograde cholangiopancreatography, ERCP, Fig. 13) or the percutaneous approach (percutaneous transhepatic cholangiography, PTC). The latter does not allow the ampulla of Vater or pancreatic duct to be visualised. MRCP is as good as ERCP at providing images of the biliary tree but has fewer complications and is the diagnostic test of choice.

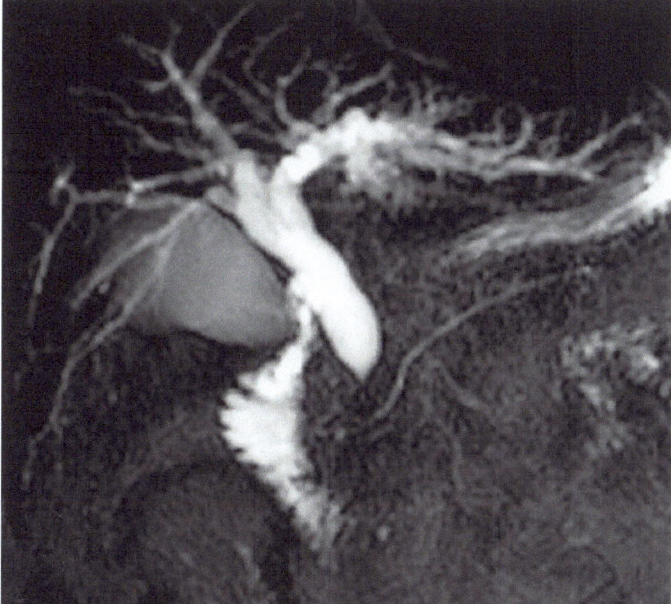

Fig. 12: MRCP showing a biliary stricture due to cholangiocarcinoma in the distal common bile duct (C).

The proximal common bile duct (B) is dilated but the pancreatic duct (P) is normal.

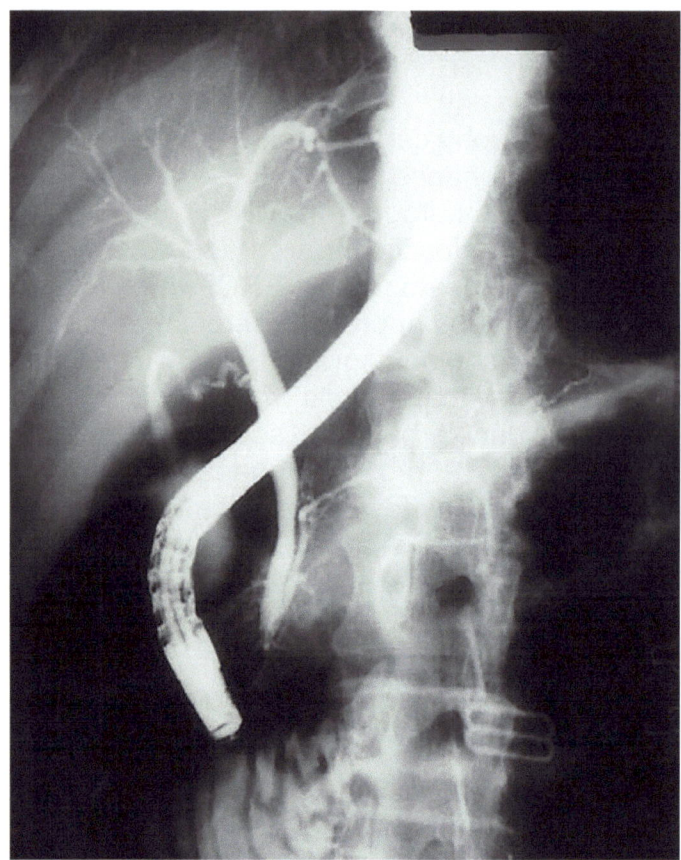

Fig. 13: ERCP showing the normal biliary (B) and pancreatic (P) duct system.
Both endoscopic and percutaneous approaches allow therapeutic interventions, such as the insertion of biliary stents across malignant bile duct strictures. The percutaneous approach is only used if it is not possible to access the bile duct endoscopically.

Histological examination:
An ultrasound-guided liver biopsy can confirm the severity of liver damage and provide aetiological information.

It is performed percutaneously with a Trucut or Menghini needle, usually through an intercostals space under local anaesthesia, or radiologically using a transjugular approach. Percutaneous liver biopsy is a relatively safe procedure if the conditions detailed in Box 7 are met, but carries a mortality of about 0.01%. The main complications are abdominal and/or shoulder pain, bleeding and biliary peritonitis. Biliary peritonitis is rare and usually occurs when a biopsy is performed in a patient with obstruction of a large bile duct. Liver biopsies can be carried out in patients with defective haemostasis if:
• The defect is corrected with fresh frozen plasma and platelet transfusion
• The biopsy is obtained by the transjugular route, *or* the procedure is conducted percutaneously under ultrasound control and the needle track is then plugged with procoagulant material.

In patients with potentially resectable malignancy, biopsy should be avoided due to the potential risk of tumour dissemination. Operative or laparoscopic liver biopsy may sometimes be valuable.

Although the pathological features of liver disease are complex, with several features occurring together, liver disorders can be broadly classified histologically into fatty liver (steatosis), hepatitis (inflammation,'grade') and cirrhosis (fibrosis, 'stage'). The use of special histological stains can help in determining aetiology.

The clinical features and prognosis of these changes are dependent on the underlying aetiology, and are discussed in the relevant sections below.

Box 7: **Conditions required for safe percutaneous liver biopsy**

Cooperative patient
• Prothrombin time < 4 secs prolonged
• Platelet count > 80 × 109/L
• Exclusion of bile duct obstruction, localised skin infection, advanced chronic obstructive pulmonary disease, marked ascites and severe anaemia.

Non-invasive markers of hepatic fibrosis

Non-invasive markers of liver fibrosis have been developed and can reduce the need for liver biopsy to assess the extent of fibrosis in some settings.

Serological markers of hepatic fibrosis, such as α2-macroglobulin, haptoglobin and routine clinical biochemistry tests, are used in the Fibrotest. The ELF (Enhanced Liver Fibrosis) serological assay uses a combination of hyaluronic acid, procollagen peptide III(PIIINP) and tissue inhibitor of metalloproteinase 1(TIMP1). These tests are good at differentiating severe fibrosis from mild scarring, but are limited in their ability to detect subtle changes. A number of non-commercial scores based on standard biochemical and anthropometric indices have also been described that provide similar levels of sensitivity and specificity (e.g. the FIB4 Score). An alternative to serological markers is transient elastography in which ultrasound-based shock waves are sent through the liver to measure liver stiffness as a surrogate for hepatic fibrosis. Once again, this test is good at differentiating severe fibrosis from mild scarring, but is limited in its ability to detect subtle changes, and validity may be affected by obesity.

Assessment of liver size:

Clinical assessment of hepatomegaly is important in diagnosing liver disease.
• Start in the right iliac fossa.
• Progress up the abdomen 2 cm with each breath (through open mouth).
• Confirm the lower border of the liver by percussion.
• Detect if smooth or irregular, tender or non-tender; ascertain shape.
• Identify the upper border by percussion.

Diseases that cause hepatomegaly can severely interfere with your liver's ability to function normally. Many of the symptoms and dangers of diseases that cause hepatomegaly relate to the inability of your liver to handle bile production and its flow, as well as impairments such as the ability to store glycogen and make important clotting factors.

According to MedlinePlus, the most common

Symptoms Associated With Hepatomegaly:

All of the symptoms associated with

hepatomegaly are serious. You should see

your doctor if you have any of the following

symptoms:

- jaundice (yellowing of the skin and eyes caused by the blockage of bile)
- fatigue
- itching
- nausea
- vomiting
- abdominal pain or fullness
- swelling of the feet and legs
- easy bruising (caused by decrease production of clotting factors)
- vomiting blood
- black tarry stools (actually blood that has been broken down in the stomach and intestines)
- shortness of breath (associated with congestive heart failure and pericarditis)
- weight loss

Nausea, vomiting (with or without blood), abdominal pain, tarry stools, and shortness of breath are medical emergencies.

What to Expect From the Doctor

A complete medical history and physical exam are the first steps to finding the reason why your liver is enlarged.

Treatment:

The underlying disorders that cause your liver to be enlarged determine your treatment options. Congestive heart failure can be treated with medications. Treatment options for liver cancer include chemotherapy, surgery, and liver transplant. Metastatic cancer is treated according to the source of the cancer. Treatment options for lymphoma depend upon the type, stage (degree of spread), and your general health.

Long-Term Consequences of Non-Treatment Failure to diagnose and treat the underlying cause of hepatomegaly can be fatal.

Prevention:

There are many common-sense measures you can take to protect your liver. Some of the things you can do are:

- Exercise caution when drinking alcohol and consider not drinking at all. Discuss your drinking habits with your doctor to see if your intake is excessive.
- Take vitamin supplements only as directed, and always discuss them with your doctor.

  Exercise caution in taking herbal supplements. Always discuss any herbs you are considering taking with your doctor. According to the MayoClinic, (2012), herbs that can damage your liver include: black cohosh, chaparral comfrey, germander, ma-huang, skullcap, kava, mistletoe, valerian, and pennyroyal
- Eat a balanced diet containing whole grains, vegetables, and fruit.
- Maintain an optimal weight.
- Stop smoking.

Inherited liver diseases

The inherited diseases are an important and probably under-diagnosed group of liver diseases. In addition to the 'classical' conditions such as haemochromatosis and Wilson's disease, the important role played by the liver in the expression of the inborn errors of metabolism should be remembered, as should the potential for genetic underpinning for intrahepatic

cholestasis.

Hemochromatosis

Definition of disease:

a condition in which the amount of total body iron is increased; the excess iron is deposited in, and causes damage to, several organs, including the liver, Hepatic abnormalities and cirrhosis, heart failure, hypogonadism, and arthritis.

Usually suspected because of elevated iron saturation or serum ferritin or a family history.

Most patients are asymptomatic; the disease is rarely recognized clinically before the fifth decade.

HFE gene mutation (usually *C282Y/C282Y*) is found in most cases.

Disease classification:

• The disease can be classified into stages:

• Stage 1: patients with the genetic disorder (positive HFE gene test) but normal iron stores.

• Stage 2: patients with the genetic disorder and elevated iron stores but no tissue/organ damage.

• Stage 3: patients with the genetic disorder with iron overload and tissue/organ damage.

• In addition, iron overload can be classified according to whether it is an inherited disorder (as in HH) or one of the many causes of secondary iron overload.

Incidence/prevalence:

It may be primary or secondary to other diseases (Box 8).

Box 8: Causes of haemochromatosis:

Primary haemochromatosis

• Hereditary haemochromatosis
• Congenital acaeruloplasminaemia
• Congenital atransferrinaemia

Secondary iron overload

• Parenteral iron-loading (e.g. repeated blood transfusion)
• Iron-loading anaemia (thalassaemia, sideroblastic anaemia, pyruvate kinase deficiency)
• Liver disease

Complex iron overload

• Juvenile haemochromatosis
• Neonatal haemochromatosis
• Alcoholic liver disease
• Porphyria cutanea tarda
• African iron overload (Bantu siderosis)

Essentials of diagnosis:

General Considerations:

Hemochromatosis is an autosomal recessive disease caused in many cases by a mutation in the *HFE* gene on chromosome 6. The HFE protein is thought to play an important role in the process by which duodenal crypt cells sense body iron stores, leading in turn to increased iron absorption from the duodenum. A decrease in the synthesis or expression of hepcidin, the principal iron regulatory hormone, is thought to be a key pathogenic factor in all forms of hemochromatosis. About 85% of persons with well established hemochromatosis are homozygous for the *C282Y* mutation. The frequency of the gene mutation averages 7% in Northern European and North American white populations, resulting in a 0.5% frequency of homozygotes(of whom 38–50% will develop biochemical evidence of iron overload but only 28% of men and 1% of women will develop clinical symptoms). By contrast, the gene mutation and hemochromatosis are uncommon in blacks and Asian-American populations. A second genetic mutation (*H63D*) may contribute to the development of iron overload in a small percentage (1.5%) of persons who are compound heterozygotes for *C282Y* and *H63D;* iron overload-related disease develops in few patients (particularly those who have a comorbidity such as diabetes mellitus and fatty liver). *H63D* homozygotes do not develop hemochromatosis but may be at increased risk for amyotrophic lateral sclerosis. Rare instances of hemochromatosis result from mutations in the genes that encode transferrin receptor 2 (*TFR2*) and ferroportin (*FPN1*). A juvenile-onset variant that is characterized by severe iron overload, cardiac dysfunction, hypogonadotropic hypogonadism, and a high mortality rate is usually linked to a mutation of a gene on chromosome 1q designated *HJV* that produces a protein called hemojuvelin or, rarely, to a mutation in the *HAMP* gene on chromosome 19 that encodes hepcidin but not to the *C282Y* mutation.

Hemochromatosis is characterized by increased accumulation of iron as hemosiderin in the liver, pancreas, heart, adrenals, testes, pituitary, and kidneys. Cirrhosis is more likely to develop in affected persons who drink alcohol excessively or have obesity-related hepatic steatosis than in those who do not. Eventually, hepatic and pancreatic insufficiency, heart failure, and hypogonadism may develop; overall mortality is increased slightly.

Heterozygotes do not develop cirrhosis in the absence of associated disorders such as viral hepatitis or NAFLD.

Clinical Findings:

A. Symptoms and Signs

The onset of clinical disease is usually after age 50 years—earlier in men than in women "over 40 years in men"; however, because of widespread liver biochemical testing and iron screening, the diagnosis is usually made long before symptoms develop. Early symptoms are nonspecific (eg: generalized weakness, fatigue, and arthralgia).

Later clinical manifestations include arthropathy (and the need for joint replacement surgery), hepatomegaly and evidence of hepatic dysfunction (late finding), skin pigmentation(combination of slate-gray due to iron and brown due to melanin, sometimes resulting in a bronze colour) especially in exposed parts, axillae, groins and genitalia: hence the term 'bronzed diabetes'., cardiac enlargement with or without heart failure or conduction defects, diabetes mellitus with its complications, and erectile dysfunction in men "loss of libido", Impotence. Interestingly, population studies have shown an increased prevalence of liver disease but not of diabetes mellitus, arthritis, or heart disease in *C282Y* homozygotes. In patients in whom cirrhosis develops, bleeding from oesophageal varices may occur, and there is a 15–20% frequency of hepatocellular carcinoma. Affected patients are at increased risk of infection with *Vibrio vulnificus, Listeria monocytogenes, Yersinia enterocolitica*, and other siderophilic organisms. The risk of porphyria cutanea tarda is increased in persons with the *C282Y* or *H63D* mutation, and *C282Y* homozygotes have twice the risk of colorectal and breast cancer than persons without the *C282Y* variant. Arthritis with chondrocalcinosis secondary to calcium pyrophosphate deposition are also common.

Cardiac failure or cardiac dysrhythmia may occur due to iron deposition in the heart. Once again, absence of this feature does not preclude the diagnosis.

•Examination findings can include cardiomegaly, hepatomegaly, testicular atrophy, skin pigmentation and arthritis.

B. Laboratory Findings:

Laboratory findings include:

1. mildly abnormal liver tests(AST, alkaline phosphatase),
2. An elevated plasma iron with > 45% transferrin saturation and an elevated serum ferritin (although a normal iron saturation or a normal ferritin does not exclude the diagnosis). Affected men are more likely than affected women to have an elevated ferritin level.

The differential diagnoses for elevated ferritin are inflammatory disease particularly chronic liver diseases due to alcohol, viral hepatitis and fatty liver disease or excess ethanol consumption for modest elevations (< 1000 µg/L). Very significant ferritin elevation can be seen in adult Still's disease.

3-Testing for *HFE* mutations is indicated in any patient with evidence of iron overload.

C. Imaging:

1-MRI and

2-CT

May show changes consistent with iron overload of the liver, and MRI can quantitate hepatic iron stores. There is also an emerging role for MRI for assessment of the degree of hepatic fibrosis. MRI has high specificity for iron overload, but poor sensitivity.

D. Liver Biopsy:

In patients who are homozygous for *C282Y*, liver biopsy is often indicated to determine whether cirrhosis is present.

Biopsy can be deferred, however, in patients in whom the serum ferritin level is 1000 mcg/L, serum AST level is normal, and hepatomegaly is absent; the likelihood of cirrhosis is low in these persons. The combination of a serum ferritin level ≥1000 mcg/L and a serum hyaluronic acid level ≥46.5 mcg/L has been reported to identify all patients with cirrhosis, with a high specificity. Liver biopsy is also indicated when iron overload is suspected even though the patient is not homozygous for *C282Y* or a *C282Y/H63D* compound heterozygote. In patients with hemochromatosis, the liver biopsy characteristically shows extensive iron deposition in hepatocytes and in bile ducts, and the hepatic iron index(HII) (μmol of iron per g dry weight of liver/age in years) — hepatic iron content per gram of liver converted to micromoles and divided by the patient's age—is generally > 1.9. Only 5% of patients with hereditary "genetic " hemochromatosis identified by screening in a primary care setting have cirrhosis. Liver biopsy allows assessment of fibrosis and distribution of iron (hepatocyte iron characteristic of haemochromatosis).

Both the C282Y and the H63D mutations can be identified by genetic testing, which is now in routine clinical use.

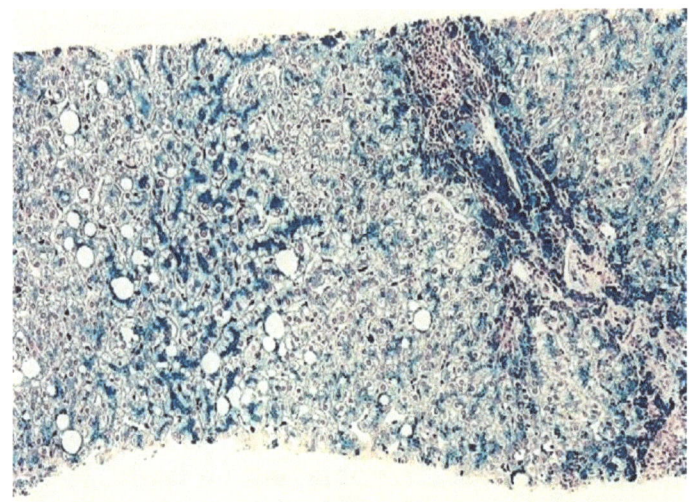

Fig. 14: Liver histology: haemochromatosis. This Perls stain shows accumulating iron within hepatocytes, which is stained blue.

There is also accumulation of large fat globules in some hepatocytes (macrovesicular steatosis). Iron also accumulates in Kupffer cells and biliary epithelial cells.

Screening:

Iron studies and *HFE* testing are recommended for all first degree family members of a proband; children of an affected person (*C282Y* homozygote) need to be screened only if the patient's spouse carries the *C282Y* or *H63D* mutation. Average-risk population screening for hemochromatosis is not recommended because the clinical penetrance of *C282Y* homozygosity and morbidity and mortality from hemochromatosis are low. Patients with otherwise unexplained chronic liver disease, chondrocalcinosis, erectile dysfunction, and type 1 diabetes mellitus (especially late-onset) should be screened for iron overload.

Screening:
• Screening tests for HH depend on the patient population being investigated.
• Despite the high prevalence of HFE gene mutations, the low disease penetrance means that routine screening of the general population is not recommended.
• Patients with abnormal liver enzymes or clinical evidence of liver disease should be screened for HH.
• Patients with a family history of HH should be screened.
• The initial screening test for HH should include serum iron studies: transferrin saturation and ferritin.
• If the transferrin saturation is greater than 45% or the ferritin is above the normal range, genetic testing for HFE mutations is recommended.
• In patients with a first degree relative with HH, iron studies and HFE genetic testing is recommended.

Liver biopsy is only indicated in asymptomatic relatives if the LFTs are abnormal and/or the serum ferritin is greater than 1000 µg/L because these features are associated with significant fibrosis or cirrhosis.

Treatment:

1-Affected patients should avoid foods rich in iron (such as red meat), alcohol, vitamin C, raw shellfish, and supplemental iron.

2-Weekly phlebotomies of 1 or 2 units (250–500 mL) of blood (each containing about 250 mg of iron) is indicated in all symptomatic patients, those with a serum ferritin level of at least 1000 mcg/L, and those with an increased fasting iron saturation and should be continued for up to 2–3 years to achieve depletion of iron stores. The hematocrit, serum iron values and hemoglobin should be monitored prior to phlebotomy to avoid anaemia (greater than 20% drop in haemoglobin). When iron store depletion is achieved (iron saturation <50% and serum ferritin level 50–100 mcg/L), phlebotomies (every 2–4 months) to maintain serum ferritin levels between 50 mcg/L and 100 mcg/L are continued until the serum iron is normal, although compliance has been reported to decrease with time; administration of a proton pump inhibitor, which reduces intestinal iron absorption, appears to decrease the maintenance phlebotomy blood volume requirement. First degree family members should be investigated, preferably by genetic screening and also by checking the plasma ferritin and iron-binding saturation. Asymptomatic disease should also be treated by venesection until the serum ferritin is normal. Pre-cirrhotic patients with HHC have a normal life expectancy, and even cirrhotic patients have a good prognosis compared with other forms of cirrhosis (three-quarters of patients are alive 5 years after diagnosis).

This is probably because liver function is well preserved at diagnosis and improves with therapy.

Screening for hepatocellular carcinoma (p. 967) is mandatory because this is the main cause of death, affecting one-third of patients with cirrhosis irrespective of therapy.

• Complications of phlebotomy include anaemia but can be avoided by monitoring haemoglobin levels prior to each phlebotomy.

3-Complications of hemochromatosis— arthropathy, diabetes mellitus, heart disease, portal hypertension, and hypopituitarism—also require treatment. Therapy includes that for cirrhosis and diabetes mellitus.

4-The chelating agent deferoxamine is indicated for patients with hemochromatosis and anaemia or in those with secondary iron overload due to thalassemia who cannot tolerate phlebotomies" it is the treatment of choice for secondary iron overload such as dyserythropoeisis syndromes (thalassemia, haemolytic anaemia)where anaemia prevents the use of phlebotomy". The drug is administered intravenously or subcutaneously in a dose of 20–40 mg/kg/d infused over 24 hours "for 5–7 days" and can mobilize 30 mg of iron per day; however, treatment is painful and time-consuming. An oral chelator, deferasirox, 20 mg/kg once daily, has been approved for treatment of iron overload due to blood transfusions, and a dose of 10 mg/kg daily may be appropriate in persons with hemochromatosis who cannot tolerate phlebotomy; however, this agent has many side effects and drug-drug interactions. Seldom required in HH.

The course of hemochromatosis is favourably altered by phlebotomy therapy. Hepatic fibrosis may regress, and in precirrhotic patients, cirrhosis may be prevented. Cardiac conduction defects and insulin requirements improve with treatment. In patients with cirrhosis, varices may reverse, and the risk of variceal bleeding declines, although the risk of hepatocellular carcinoma persists, joint pain is less predictable and can improve or worsen after iron removal. Diabetes mellitus does not resolve after venesection. In the past, liver transplantation for advanced cirrhosis associated with severe iron overload, including hemochromatosis, was reported to lead to survival rates that were lower than those for other types of liver disease because of cardiac complications and an increased risk of infections, but since 1997,post transplant survival rates have been excellent.

When to Refer:

• For liver biopsy.
• For initiation of therapy.

Hereditary haemochromatosis:

• There is no universally accepted definition of HH but it is essentially an inherited condition leading to increased total body iron.
• The prevalence of HH defined by HFE gene polymorphisms varies according to population but is as high as 1 in 140 for C282Y homozygosity in people of Northern European ancestry and 1 in 330 in a racially mixed population.
The frequency of the C282Y allele is as high as 12.5% in Ireland.
• C282Y homozygosity accounts for approximately 80% of inherited iron overload syndromes, with 5% accounted for by C282Y and H63D heterozygosity. The remaining 15% likely have mutations in other genes involved in iron absorption and metabolism.
In hereditary haemochromatosis (HHC), iron is deposited throughout the body and

total body iron may reach 20–60 g (normally 4 g). The important organs involved are the liver, pancreatic islets, endocrine glands and heart. In the liver, iron deposition occurs first in the periportal hepatocytes, extending later to all hepatocytes.
The gradual development of fibrous septa leads to the formation of irregular nodules, and finally regeneration results in macronodular cirrhosis. An excess of liver iron can occur in alcoholic cirrhosis but this is mild by comparison with haemochromatosis.

Pathophysiology:

The disease is caused by increased absorption of dietary iron and is inherited as an autosomal recessive trait. Approximately 90% of patients are homozygous for a single-point mutation resulting in a cysteine to tyrosine substitution at position 282 (C282Y) in the HFE protein, which has structural and functional similarity to the HLA proteins. The mechanisms by which HFE regulates iron absorption are unclear. However, it is believed that HFE normally interacts with the transferrin receptor in the basolateral membrane of intestinal epithelial cells. In HHC, it is thought that the lack of functional HFE causes a defect in uptake of transferrin-associated iron, leading to up-regulation of enterocyte iron-specific divalent metal transporters and excessive iron absorption. A histidine to aspartic acid mutation at position 63 (H63D) in HFE causes a less severe form of haemochromatosis that is most commonly found in patients who are compound heterozygotes also carrying a C282Y mutated allele.

Fewer than 50% of C282Y homozygotes will develop clinical features of haemochromatosis; therefore other factors must also be important. HHC may promote accelerated liver disease in patients with alcohol excess or hepatitis C infection. Iron loss in menstruation and pregnancy can delay the onset of HHC in females.

OVERALL BOTTOM LINE

• HH is an autosomal recessive disease caused by mutations in the HFE gene leading to increased iron absorption and deposition of iron in various organs, including the liver.

• It is the most common hereditary disorder in White people with a prevalence as high as 1 in 140 individuals in some studies although phenotypic expression is much less common.

• It typically presents as asymptomatic elevation in iron studies but can present in middle age with abnormal liver enzymes and hepatomegaly as well as arthralgias, loss of libido, diabetes and heart failure due to iron deposition in other organs.

• The diagnosis relies on demonstration of elevated body iron stores with a high iron saturation and ferritin. Testing for HFE gene mutations and hepatic iron content on liver biopsy can also be helpful.

• Treatment is based on depletion of iron through phlebotomy and improves survival and can even reverse cirrhosis in selected patients.

Background:

Economic impact

• The economic impact of HH is unclear. Despite the high prevalence of the disorder, the low phenotypic expression and simplicity of treatment would suggest a minimal economic impact compared with other causes of chronic liver disease.

Etiology:

• There are several genetic defects that have been identified in HH.

• The commonest genetic defect is closely linked to the HLA-A3 locus on the short arm of chromosome 6. In 1996, two missense mutations were identified on a candidate gene and termed the HLA-H or HFE gene.

• Substitution of tyrosine for cysteine at amino acid position 282 (C282Y) of the HFE gene product is the commonest with C282Y homozygotes accounting for 80–85% of all HH patients. Substitution of histidine for aspartate at position 63 (H63D) and serine substituted for cysteine at position 65 (S65C) make up the other two commonly identified mutations but are rarely seen in iron overload unless associated with C282Y in a compound heterozygote.

•Several other mutations in genes encoding for a variety of other proteins involved in iron regulation (hepcidin, ferroportin, hemojuvelin, and transferrin receptor 2, ceruloplasmin) probably play a role in HH in the absence of HFE gene mutations.

Pathology/pathogenesis:

• In normal individuals, 1 mg of iron is lost daily through skin, sweat and the gastrointestinal tract and is replaced by 1 mg absorbed through duodenal enterocytes, a process regulated by iron stores.

• In HH, failure of this regulatory mechanism leads to absorption of several milligrams of iron daily which overcomes the normal iron loss. After the increased need for iron in childhood and adolescence abates, iron stores gradually increase at a rate of approximately 1 g a year (less in women due to menstruation, pregnancy and lactation). By middle age 20–30 g of excess iron has been deposited in several organs leading to the clinical manifestations.

• Liver damage in HH is thought to be related to iron-dependent oxidative processes which damage several cell functions initiating a cascade of cytokines that ultimately lead to fibrosis.

• The function of the HFE gene protein is still unclear but it is structurally similar to major histocompatibility complex class-1 proteins and can bind to transferrin receptors (1 and 2). The resulting complex may have a role in sensing iron on the hepatocyte cell membrane and/or affecting hepcidin expression, and may be involved in iron uptake by duodenal enterocytes.

• Hepcidin appears to be the most important peptide in iron regulation. It is made in hepatocytes and secreted into the circulation where it encounters ferroportin on macrophages and enterocytes. The hepcidin binds to ferroportin which is internalized and inhibits iron release. Excess iron induces hepcidin expression while iron deficiency decreases it.

• HFE gene mutations decrease hepcidin expression leading to up-regulation of ferroportin levels in enterocytes and an increase in intestinal iron absorption.

Prevention:

CLINICAL PEARLS

• No interventions have been demonstrated to prevent the development of the disease.
• By definition, HH is a genetic disease so cannot be prevented. However, treatment ideally should be started in asymptomatic patients prior to clinical evidence of the disease.

Diagnosis:

CLINICAL PEARLS

• Due to the increased awareness of HH and the availability of genetic testing, approximately 75% of patients are asymptomatic at presentation.
• Laboratory testing for HH is usually prompted by the finding of abnormal liver enzymes. The initial evaluation includes demonstration of elevated iron stores based on an iron saturation of greater than 45% and an elevated ferritin.
• HFE gene testing is appropriate for patients with elevated iron studies.
• Liver biopsy and hepatic iron content are helpful in certain cases where the diagnosis is in doubt and to assess the degree of fibrosis.
• Imaging can be helpful if cirrhosis is suspected and newer MRI techniques can demonstrate increased hepatic iron content.

Differential diagnosis:

Differential diagnosis	Features
Other causes of liver disease/cirrhosis	History and physical examination may be similar. Iron studies can be elevated in cirrhosis (particularly alcoholic liver disease). Genetic testing should differentiate from HH
Heart failure/congestive hepatopathy	History and physical examination may be similar. Iron studies and imaging should differentiate from HH

Typical presentation:
• The typical presentation of HH is with elevated iron studies drawn because of abnormal liver tests or on routine screening.
• Occasionally, the patient presents for testing because of a family history of HH.
• Advanced disease with fatigue, arthralgias, loss of libido, diabetes, skin hyperpigmentation ("bronze diabetes"), and symptoms and signs of heart failure has become very uncommon.

Clinical diagnosis.
History:
• The typical patient with HH will be asymptomatic. However, it is important to enquire about fatigue, weakness,

abdominal discomfort (particularly RUQ), arthralgias (particularly second and third metacarpophalangeal joints), impotence, loss of libido, skin changes and symptoms associated with heart failure and diabetes such as weight gain, ankle edema, chest pain and shortness of breath.

Physical examination:

• The physical examination in HH should look for stigmata of chronic liver disease if cirrhosis is suspected. Clinical signs include hepatomegaly, testicular atrophy, arthritis and skin pigmentation.

• Patients can have heart failure with cardiomegaly, pulmonary edema and fluid overload. Conduction abnormalities such as sick sinus syndrome can rarely be seen.

Useful clinical decision rules and calculators

• The serum ferritin level is a useful test to exclude iron overload in HH and also can predict the degree of fibrosis or cirrhosis.

• A normal ferritin essentially excludes iron overload in HH.

• A level below 1000 µg/L usually excludes cirrhosis while a level greater than 1000 µg/L with elevated liver enzymes (ALT or AST) and platelets below 200 × 109/L strongly suggests cirrhosis(in C282Y homozygotes).

Laboratory diagnosis:

List of diagnostic tests:

• All patients suspected of having HH should have iron studies including a transferrin saturation and serum ferritin.

• The test can be repeated if only mildly elevated and ideally the patient should be fasting.
• If the transferrin saturation is >45% and/or the ferritin is abnormal (>300 µg/L in men, >200 µg/L in women), HFE genetic testing should be ordered.
• HFE genetic testing should be performed on first degree relatives of HH patients.
• Liver biopsy is not required to make the diagnosis but is helpful in determining the severity of liver disease.
• Some experts suggest that C282Y homozygous patients with normal ALT/AST, elevated transferring saturation but ferritin <1000 µg/L does not require liver biopsy and should proceed directly to treatment.
• The HII and HIC were useful tests before the advent of HFE genetic testing. An HII of >71 µmol/g dry liver is indicative of hepatic iron overload. The HIC is the HII divided by the patient's age in years. An HIC ≥0.9 was taken as good evidence of phenotypic HH but at least 30–50% of C282Y homozygotes does not have elevated iron studies and hence will not have an elevated HIC. These tests should be reserved for situations where iron studies might indicate iron overload but genetic testing is negative.
List of imaging techniques:
• Imaging is helpful in HH to assess for advanced fibrosis/cirrhosis.
• CT but particularly MRI scanning can document the hepatic iron content with some accuracy using T2-weighted or R2

(mean liver proton transverse relaxation rate) images.
• The risk of HCC in HH patients is approximately 3–4% per year in patients with cirrhosis.
Hence, patients with HH and advanced fibrosis/cirrhosis should be screened every 6 months with imaging (US) and AFP. CT or MRI can be used to follow up in certain situations and to confirm findings on US.
Potential pitfalls/common errors made regarding diagnosis of disease.
• Being C282Y homozygous does not necessarily lead to phenotypic HH. Hence, HFE genetic testing should only be performed in individuals with elevated iron studies or first degree relatives of HH patients.
Table of treatment
Prevention/management of complications
CLINICAL PEARLS
• Phlebotomy in patients with HH should be initiated prior to the onset of symptoms and before evidence of organ damage.
• In symptomatic patients, phlebotomy can be expected to improve fatigue, skin changes, insulin requirement in diabetics, cardiac function and reversal of fibrosis in some patients. It does not improve arthropathy or testicular atrophy.
• In HH patients without cirrhosis, removal of iron eliminates the risk of HCC.
Special Populations:
Pregnancy
• Although unusual, pregnancy can occur in

patients with HH and can remove up to 1 g of iron.

If iron overload is present, iron supplements should not be given during pregnancy. Treatment with phlebotomy should be deferred until after pregnancy.

Prognosis:

CLINICAL PEARLS

• Patients with HH and cirrhosis are at risk for decompensated liver disease and HCC.

• In patients with HH without cirrhosis, phlebotomy improves survival.

• Patients with cirrhosis are still at risk of HCC even after adequate phlebotomy.

Natural history of untreated disease

• Without treatment HH patients are at risk for decompensated cirrhosis and HCC although the actual risk is difficult to quantify due to lack of disease penetrance of C282Y homozygotes.

• HCC is a major cause of death in HH patients with cirrhosis.

Prognosis for treated patients

• Patients with HH who undergo phlebotomy prior to symptoms or cirrhosis have a normal life expectancy.

Follow-up tests and monitoring

• The serum ferritin level is used to monitor HH patients on treatment. A target level of 50–100 µg/L is optimal.

Section 9: Evidence

Type of evidence	Title, date	Comment
Cohort study	Long-term survival analysis in hereditary hemochromatosis. Gastroenterology 1991;101:368	Demonstrated that in HH with cirrhosis survival was poor. Phlebotomy prior to cirrhosis leads to long-term survival similar to the general population
Cohort study	Long-term survival in patients with hereditary hemochromatosis. Gastroenterology 1996;110:1107	Demonstrated that iron overload in HH is associated with worse outcome and phlebotomy essentially prevents this

• Patients with HH and cirrhosis should undergo imaging every 6 months as surveillance for HCC.

Secondary haemochromatosis:

Many conditions, including chronic haemolytic disorders, sideroblastic anaemia, other conditions requiring multiple blood transfusion (generally over 50 L), porphyria cutanea tarda, dietary iron overload and occasionally alcoholic cirrhosis, are associated with widespread secondary siderosis. The features are similar to primary haemochromatosis, but the history and clinical findings point to the true diagnosis. Some patients are heterozygotes for the *HFE* gene and this may contribute to the development of iron overload.

Wilson's disease

Wilson's disease (hepatolenticular degeneration) is a rare but important autosomal recessive disorder of copper metabolism caused by a variety of mutations in a copper-transporting adenosine triphosphatase *ATP7B* gene on chromosome 13(locus: 13q14.3-q21.1), which codes for an ATP-dependent copper export pump. Total body copper is increased, with excess copper deposited in, and causing oxidative damage of hepatic mitochondria, in liver and several organs. It most commonly presents with isolated hepatic, neurological or psychiatric manifestations but multisystem involvement is not uncommon.

Pathophysiology

Normally, dietary copper is absorbed from the stomach and proximal small intestine, and is rapidly taken into the liver, where it is stored and incorporated into caeruloplasmin, which is secreted into the blood. The accumulation of excessive copper in the body is ultimately prevented by its excretion, the most important route is being via bile. In Wilson's disease, there is almost always a failure of synthesis of caeruloplasmin; however, some 5% of patients have a normal circulating caeruloplasmin concentration and this is not the primary pathogenic defect. The amount of copper in the body at birth is normal, but thereafter it increases steadily; the organs most affected are the liver, basal ganglia of the brain, eyes" cornea", kidneys and skeleton. The *ATP7B* gene encodes a member of the copper transporting P-type adenosine triphosphatase family, which functions to export copper from various cell types. At least 200 different mutations have been described. Most cases are compound heterozygotes with two different mutations in *ATP7B.* Attempts to correlate the genotype with the mode of presentation and clinical course have not shown any consistent patterns. The large number of culprit mutations means that, in contrast to haemochromatosis, genetic diagnosis is not routine in Wilson's disease, although it may have a role in screening families following identification of the genotype in an index patient. Usually occurs in persons under age 40.

Serum ceruloplasmin, the plasma copper-carrying protein, is low.

Urinary excretion of copper and hepatic copper concentration is high.

The frequency of carriers of the ATP7B mutation is about 0.6–1%.

 Economic impact

• Given the low prevalence of WD, its economic impact is not great.

• WD and alpha-1 antitrypsin deficiency disease combined account for less than 5% of liver transplant procedures in the USA according to Organ Procurement and Transplantation Network data.

General Considerations:

The worldwide prevalence is about 30 per

million populations. Siblings of a WD patient have a 1 in 4 risk of disease; children of a WD patient have one in 200 risk.

Most patients are compound heterozygotes (i.e., carry two different mutations). Over 500 mutations in the Wilson disease gene have been identified. The *H1069Q* mutation accounts for 37–63% of disease alleles in populations of Northern European descent. Consanguinity increases prevalence in some regions (e.g. Crete, Sardinia, Japanese islands).

Clinical features:

Symptoms usually arise between the ages of 5 and 45 years. Hepatic disease occurs predominantly in childhood and early adolescence, although it can present in adults in their fifties. Neurological damage causes basal ganglion syndromes and dementia, which tends to present in later adolescence. These features can occur alone or simultaneously. Other manifestations include renal tubular damage and osteoporosis, but these are rarely presenting features.

Liver disease

Episodes of acute hepatitis, sometimes recurrent, can occur, especially in children, and may progress to fulminant liver failure. The latter is characterised by the liberation of free copper into the blood stream, causing massive haemolysis and renal tubulopathy. Hepatic involvement may range from elevated liver biochemical tests (although the alkaline phosphatase may be low) to cirrhosis and portal hypertension Chronic hepatitis can also develop insidiously and eventually present with established cirrhosis; liver failure and portal hypertension may supervene. The possibility of Wilson's disease should be considered in any patient under the age of 40 presenting with recurrent acute hepatitis or chronic liver disease of unknown cause, especially when accompanied by haemolysis. In a patient with acute liver failure, the diagnosis of Wilson disease is suggested by an alkaline phosphatase (in units/L)-to-total bilirubin (in mg/dL) ratio <4 and an AST-to-ALT ratio > 2.2.

Neurological disease Clinical features include a variety of extrapyramidal features, particularly tremor, choreoathetosis, dystonia, parkinsonism and dementia. The neurologic manifestations of Wilson disease are related to basal ganglia dysfunction and include an akinetic-rigid syndrome similar to parkinsonism, pseudo sclerosis with tremor, ataxia, and a dystonic syndrome and mask-like facies. Dysarthria, dysphagia, incoordination, and spasticity are common. Migraines, insomnia, and seizures have been reported. Psychiatric features include behavioural and personality changes and emotional liability and may precede characteristic neurologic features. About a third of patients

Manifest a neuropsychiatric finding: emotional liability, anxiety or even psychosis.

Unusual clumsiness for age may be an early symptom. Neurological disease typically develops after the onset of liver disease and can be prevented by effective treatment started following diagnosis in the liver disease phase. This increases the importance of diagnosis in the liver phase beyond just allowing effective management of liver disease. The diagnosis should always be considered in any child or young adult with hepatitis, splenomegaly with hypersplenism, Coomb negative haemolytic anaemia, portal hypertension, and neurologic or psychiatric abnormalities.

Kayser–Fleischer rings:
These constitute the most important single clinical clue to the diagnosis and can be seen in 60% of adults with Wilson's disease (less often in children but almost always in neurological Wilson's disease), albeit sometimes only by slit-lamp examination. Kayser–Fleischer rings are characterised by greenish-brown discoloration of the corneal margin appearing first at the upper periphery which represents fine pigmented granular deposits in Descemet membrane in the cornea (see p. 922) (Figure 16–4). The ring is usually most marked at the superior and inferior poles of the cornea. It is sometimes seen with the naked eye and is readily detected by slit lamp examination. It may be absent in patients with hepatic manifestations only but is usually present in those with neuropsychiatric disease. They disappear with treatment.

Renal calculi, aminoaciduria, renal tubular

acidosis, hypoparathyroidism, infertility, and haemolytic anaemia may occur in patients with Wilson disease.

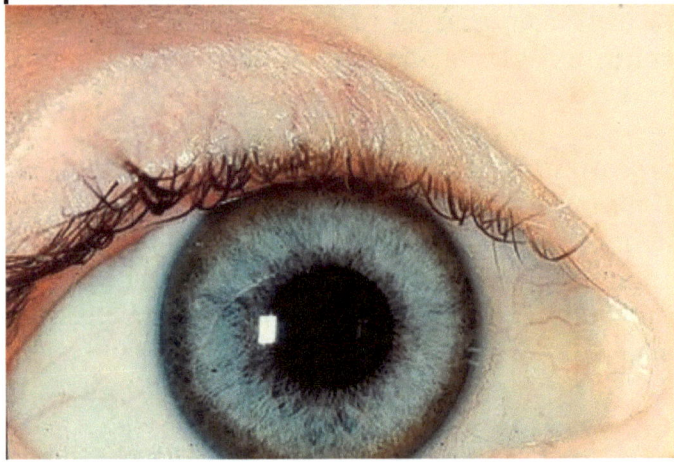

Figure 15: Brownish Kayser-Fleischer ring at the rim of the cornea in a patient with Wilson disease.

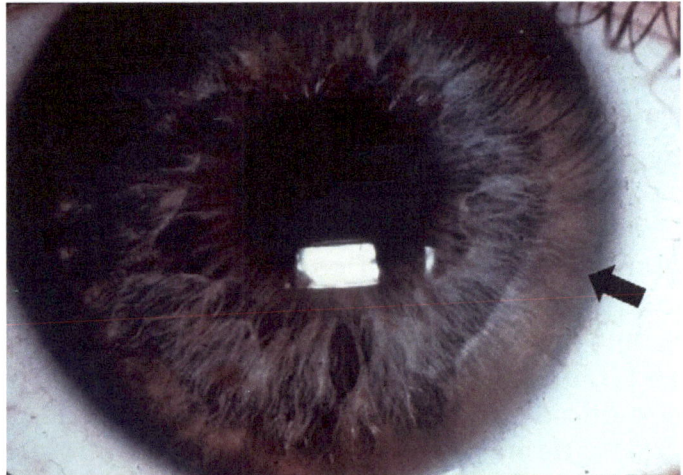

Figure 16: KF ring. Aberrant copper deposition in WD may be detected as a brownish ring (KF ring) in the

limbus zone of the eye (black arrow). A slit-lamp examination may be needed to detect KF rings in early stage
disease. Not all individuals with WD will have KF rings.

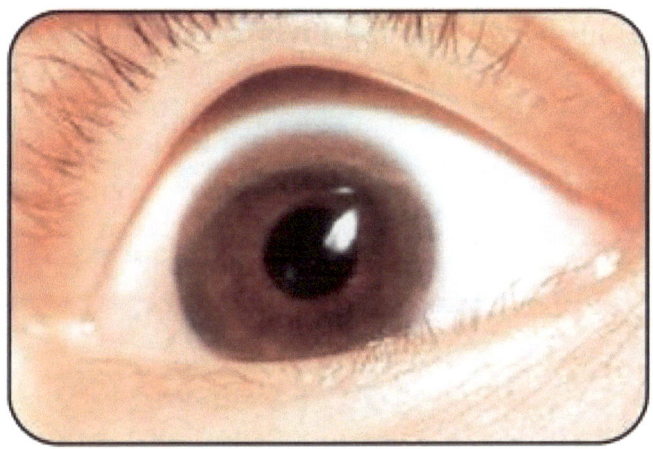

Fig 17: Kayser–Fleischer rings in Wilson's disease

Screening:

• Genetic, ophthalmologic and biochemical tests are used to screen for WD. It is not cost effective to screen the general population due to the large number of known mutations and the rarity of the disease. However, first degree relatives of any patient with WD should be screened since early treatment can prevent disease onset.

Differential diagnosis:

Differential diagnosis	Features
Drug or toxin-induced hepatitis/liver failure	A thorough history is needed to rule out hepatotoxicity due to medications and toxin exposure. Be aware that multiple products contain acetaminophen
Viral hepatitis	
AIH	History of travel, transfusion, needle sharing, or tattoos. Positive viral serological markers
NAFLD	
Other psychiatric disorder	Characterized by serum autoantibodies and interface hepatitis on the biopsy Normal serum ceruloplasmin and urinary copper levels. No KF rings Normal serum ceruloplasmin and urinary copper levels. No KF

	rings. Diagnose by DSM IV

Investigations:

1-A low serum caeruloplasmin (<20 mg/dL [200 mg/L]; <5 mg/dL [50 mg/L] is diagnostic) is the best single laboratory clue to the diagnosis. However, advanced liver failure from any cause can reduce the serum caeruloplasmin, and occasionally it is normal in Wilson's disease. A normal serum ceruloplasmin level does not exclude WD. Other features of disordered copper metabolism should therefore be sought; these include

2-a high free serum copper concentration,

3-a high urine copper excretion of greater than 0.6 µmol/24 hrs (38 µg/24 hrs) and a very high hepatic copper content.

4-Measuring 24-hour urinary copper excretion whilst giving D-penicillamine is a useful confirmatory test; more than 25 µmol/24 hrs is considered diagnostic of Wilson's disease.

In equivocal cases (when the serum ceruloplasmin level is normal), the diagnosis may require demonstration of a rise in urinary copper after a penicillamine challenge, although the test has been validated only in children.

5- Elevated hepatic copper concentration (> 250 mcg/g of dry liver).

However, increased urinary copper and a low serum ceruloplasmin level (by a standard immunologic assay) are neither completely sensitive nor specific for Wilson disease, but an enzymatic assay for ceruloplasmin appears to be more accurate.

Liver biopsy may show acute or chronic hepatitis or cirrhosis the liver biopsy features of WD are non-specific. WD can easily be confused with the histologic features of either autoimmune hepatitis or NASH. Early findings may include micro- and macrovesicular steatosis, glycogenated nuclei and portal fibrosis. Mallory bodies may be present.

MRI of the brain may show evidence of increased basal ganglia, brainstem, and cerebellar copper even early in the course of the disease. MRI of the brain may show widespread lesions in putamen, globus pallidus, caudate and thalamus. These lesions show high signal intensity on T2-weighted images and low intensity on T1.

If available, molecular analysis of *ATP7B* mutations can be diagnostic or haplotype analysis.

6-Serum LFTs: generally increased ALT and AST levels are present in WD, but they are neither sensitive nor specific. A lower than expected AP is common. A decreased uric acid level is common. Those with severe disease may have a direct hyperbilirubinemia or an indirect hyperbilirubinemia if haemolysis is present.

Prevention:

Low copper diet and zinc or chelation therapy may prevent disease onset.

Management:

Early in the treatment phase, restriction of dietary copper (shellfish, organ foods, nuts, mushrooms, and chocolate) may be of value.

For patients who are asymptomatic without cirrhosis, zinc alone is the treatment of choice.

The copper-binding agent, penicillamine, is the drug of choice. The dose given must be sufficient to produce cupriuresis and most patients require 1.5 g/day (range 1–4 g) in divided doses taken 1 h before or 2 h after food). The dose can be reduced once the disease is in remission but treatment must continue for life, even through pregnancy. Care must be taken to ensure that re-accumulation of copper does not occur. Abrupt discontinuation of treatment must be avoided because this may precipitate acute liver failure. Oral pyridoxine, 50 mg per week, is added, since penicillamine is an antimetabolite of this vitamin. Toxic effects occur in one-third of patients and include rashes, protein-losing nephropathy, lupus-like syndrome and bone marrow depression. If these do occur, trientine dihydrochloride (1.2–2.4 g/day) 250–500 mg three times a day and zinc acetate or zinc gluconate (50 mg 3 times daily) are potential alternatives, interferes with intestinal absorption of copper, promotes fecal copper excretion, and has been used as first-line therapy in presymptomatic or pregnant patients and those with neurologic disease and as maintenance therapy after decoppering with a chelating agent, but adverse gastrointestinal effects often lead to discontinuation and its long-term efficacy and safety (including a risk of hepatotoxicity) have been questioned. Ammonium tetrathiomolybdate• It should always be taken either 1 hour before or 2 hours after the meal , which complexes copper in the intestinal tract, has shown promise as initial therapy for neurologic Wilson disease.

Treatment should continue indefinitely. The doses of penicillamine and trientine should be reduced during pregnancy.

Supplemental vitamin E, an antioxidant, has been recommended but not rigorously studied. Once the serum nonceruloplasmin copper level is within the normal range (50–150 mcg/L), the dose of chelating agent can be reduced to the minimum necessary for maintaining that level. The prognosis is good in patients who are effectively treated before liver or brain damage has occurred. Liver transplantation is indicated for fulminant liver failure or for advanced cirrhosis with liver failure. The value of liver transplantation in severe neurological Wilson's disease is unclear. Prognosis is excellent, provided treatment is started before there is irreversible damage. Siblings and children of patients with Wilson's disease must be investigated and treatment should be given to all affected individuals, even if they are asymptomatic.

When to Refer

All patients with Wilson disease should be referred for

diagnosis and treatment.

When to Admit

• Acute liver failure.
• Gastrointestinal bleeding.
• Stage 3–4 hepatic encephalopathy.
• Worsening kidney function.
• Severe hyponatremia.
• Profound hypoxia.

Potential future therapies include isolated hepatocyte transplantation and gene therapy.

If a patient diagnosed with autoimmune hepatitis does not respond to steroids always keepWD in mind.

Treatment	Comment
Conservative	• Dietary modifications: foods rich in copper like chocolate, shellfish, nuts should be avoided
Medical: Chelators • D-penicillamine: 1000–1500 mg/day in 2–4 divided doses	• Antioxidants: vitamin E • Adverse affects include: sensitivity reaction marked by

	rash, neutropenia, and lymphadenopathy; nephrotoxicity; bone marrow depression; and neurological deterioration • Starting with a low initial dosage of 250–500 mg/day and gradually increase over 4–6 weeks may limit adverse reactions
• Trientine: Initiation phase: 750–1500 mg/day in 2–3 divided doses Maintenance dose: 750–1000 mg/day In 2–3 divided doses • Ammonium tetrathiomolybdate	• Take either 1 hour before or 2 hours after the meal • Pregnant women, children and the malnourished should take vitamin B6 supplements • Monitoring of urine protein and blood cell counts needs to be done regularly
Non-chelator • Zinc: dosage of 150 mg is administered in adults and 75 mg in small children is	• It should always be taken either 1 hour before or 2 hours after the meal • Efficacy similar to

administered in three divided doses Combination therapy	D-penicillamine but has the benefit of fewer side effects
	• Preferred for those with predominantly neurological symptoms where available
• Zinc + chelator Dialysis, hemofiltration, or plasmapheresis	
	• Take either 1 hour before or 2 hours after the meal. • Adverse effects: immune suppression, pancreatitis • To check the efficacy of treatment, 24-hour urinary copper excretion is measured. The level should be high for chelator therapy and low for zinc therapy • There should be a 3–4 hour interval between doses
Surgical: • Liver transplantation	• Emergency treatment for copper

	overload in fulminant liver failure • For patients with fulminant liver failure or decompensated cirrhosis who fail to respond to medical therapy

CLINICAL PEARLS

• Chelating agents may cause worsening of neurologic symptoms when therapy is initiated.
Gradually increasing the dose of these agents may help in decreasing this problem.

• Asymptomatic individuals should be encouraged to continue zinc treatment lifelong.

• Those that become asymptomatic on treatment should not stop treatment, but can be switched to zinc alone. Zinc may be considered in patients who cannot tolerate first line agents or who have worsening of neuropsychiatric disease with the chelating agents.

• Urinary copper testing can be performed to detect suspected non-compliance with treatment.

• D-penicillamine inactivates pyridoxine so small doses of pyridoxine (25 mg/day) should be given with D-penicillamine.

Special Populations
Pregnancy

• Treatment must be continued during the entire course of pregnancy. Both chelators and zinc have been associated with favourable outcome. However, due to the safety profile of zinc and trientine, they are preferred over penicillamine. Chelators should be used at the lowest effective dose.
Children:
• The treatment options remain the same although dose reductions are required. Zinc or trientine are the safer option.
Follow-up tests and monitoring
• Perform a physical examination, 24-hour urinary copper excretion assay, CBC count, urinalysis, serum ceruloplasmin level and renal and liver function tests on a biweekly basis for first 2 months, followed by monthly visits for the next 2 or 3 months and after that every 6 months.
• In patients with a KF ring a yearly slit lamp examination should be performed.
• Patients should be told about warning symptoms of worsening liver or neurological disease.
• After dosage adjustment of a chelator, a 24-hour urinary copper measurement should be performed.
• If non-compliance with chelator therapy is suspected, measure the level of non-ceruloplasmin bound copper which will be increased in those who are non-compliant.

Index

Box no:	comment
1	**Causes of change in liver size Large liver (hepatomegaly)**
2	**Aims of investigations in patients with suspected liver disease**
3	**Hepatitic 'and' cholestatic'/'obstructive' Liver function tests.**
4	**Drugs that increase levels of gamma-glutamyltransferase**
5	**Chronic liver disease screen**
6	**How to identify the cause of LFT abnormality**
7	**Conditions required for safe percutaneous liver biopsy**
8	**Causes of haemochromatosis:**

A table show box number and comment about each box.

Figure no	comment	page
1	Congestive Heart Failure (CHF)	14
2	Cirrhosis.	15
3	Hepatitis.	15
4	Liver Cancer.	16
5	Hyperlipidemia.	16
6	Familial Combined Hyperlipidemia	17
7	Hyperlipoproteinemia Type IV	18
8	Adult-Onset Still's Disease	19
9	Hyperlipoproteinemia	20
10	Ultrasound showing a stone in the gallbladder. Stone (arrow) with acoustic shadow (S).	31
11	CT scan in a patient with cirrhosis.	32
12	MRCP showing a biliary stricture due to cholangiocarcinoma in the distal common bile duct (C).	33
13	ERCP showing the normal biliary (B) and pancreatic (P) duct system.	34
14	Liver histology	48

15	Brownish Kayser-Fleischer ring at the rim of the cornea in a patient with Wilson disease.	71
16	KF ring. Aberrant copper deposition in WD may be detected as a brownish ring (KF ring) in the limbus zone of the eye (black arrow). A slit-lamp examination may be needed to detect KF rings in early stage disease. Not all individuals with WD will have KF rings.	72
17	Kayser–Fleischer rings in Wilson's disease	73

A table show figure number, a comment and page number of each figure.

References of the book:

1-Current Medical Diagnosis and Treatment 2014.
2-Davidson's Principles and Practice of Medicine.
3-Mount Sinai Expert Guides – Hepatology
4-What causes liver enlarged? 15 possible conditions .Medically Reviewed by George Krucik, MD, MBA. Written by Verneda Lights.

Article Sources:

Enlarged Liver Causes. (2012, April 14). Mayo Clinic. Retrieved July 13, 2012, from http://www.mayoclinic.com/health/enlarged-liver/DS00638/DSECTION=causes

Enlarged Liver, Prevention. (2012, April 14). Mayo Clinic. Retrieved July 13, 2012, from http://www.mayoclinic.com/health/enlarged-liver/DS00638/DSECTION=prevention

Hepatomegaly. (2012, June 28). *MedlinePlus Medical Encyclopaedia,* National Library of Medicine – National Institutes of Health. Retrieved July 13, 2012, fromhttp://www.nlm.nih.gov/medlineplus/ency/article/003275.htm

Wolf, D. C. (1990). Chapter 94 Evaluation of the Size, Shape, and Consistency of the Liver. National Centre for Biotechnology Information (NCBI) Bookshelf. Retrieved July 13, 2012, from http://www.ncbi.nlm.nih.gov/books/NBK421/

About the Author

Dr / Osama Ahmed Bahudila doctor and author born in a charming town called Aden in the most beautiful country called Yemen on the twentieth of October, one thousand nine hundred and seventy-two father of five sons, Nooran , Abu Bakr, Alaa, Lena and Abdul Rahman made them God worthy successor to the best predecessor, spent most of his life in Aden where he completed most of the stages of primary and secondary school in the various schools of the province of Aden, where compulsory service spent in the field of teaching in one of the schools to reconcile after that to get a scholarship to complete his university education in the field of medicine and surgery in one of the nearby Arab countries to study there until his graduation in the year two thousand and two of the Nativity in the field of General Medicine and surgery, return to the homeland after that to work in the province of Marib as director of the hospital rural cree, which was under construction to stay in the province for a period of four years of arduous full complement then graduate studies in the field of Internal Medicine, where he completed his studies in this area specialization before moving to work in Saudi Arabia, where he worked in one of the clinics there and then returned to the homeland and still works so far in the Health and Population Office of the of the governorate of Marib/ Yemen.

The author facebook page is:

https://www.facebook.com/osama.bahudaila

The author account on twitter is:

https://twitter.com/osamaahmedbahud

The author account on google is:

https://plus.google.com/u/0/+Osamabahudila

The author account on Amazon.com :

http://www.amazon.com/s/ref=dp_byline_sr_book_1?ie=UTF8&text=Dr+osama+ahmed+bahudila&search-alias=books&field-author=Dr+osama+ahmed+bahudila&sort=relevancerank

The author youtube channel is:

https://www.youtube.com/channel/UCAQH5WoQdSzZLTWHGXXiGWw

More books from the Author

1-Notes and Jokes Doctor in the Kingdom published in December 6, 2014 at Amazon .com at this link: http://www.amazon.com/Notes-Jokes-Doctor-Kingdom Bahudila/dp/1505351480/ref=sr_1_7?s=books&ie=UTF8&qid=1441592845&sr=1-7

2-Notes and Jokes Doctor in The Kingdom: A collection of true stories (Arabic Edition) (Arabic) Paperback – January 3, 2015 at this link: http://www.amazon.com/Notes-Jokes-Doctor-Kingdom-collection/dp/1505919797/ref=sr_1_9?s=books&ie=UTF8&qid=1441593139&sr=1-9

3-Doctor Of Chieftains: A collection of true stories Paperback – January 13, 2015 at this link: http://www.amazon.com/Doctor-Chieftains-collection-true-stories/dp/1507540868/ref=sr_1_10?s=books&ie=UTF8&qid=1441593393&sr=1-10

4-A Song Penned By Alrahman: Aden (Arabic Edition) (Arabic) Paperback – April 19, 2015 at this link : http://www.amazon.com/Song-Penned-Alrahman-AdenArabic/dp/1511786345/ref=sr_1_3?s=books&ie=UTF8&qid=1441595872&sr=1-3

5-A Song Penned By Alrahman: Aden Paperback – April 21, 2015
At this link:
http://www.amazon.com/Song-Penned-Alrahman-Aden/dp/1511811056/ref=sr_1_4?s=books&ie=UTF8&qid=1441596023&sr=1-4

6-Une chanson ecrite par Arrahman: Aden (French

Edition) (French) Paperback – April 23 at this link:
http://www.amazon.com/Une-chanson-ecrite-par-Arrahman/dp/1511848057/ref=sr_1_5?s=books&ie=UTF8&qid=1441596130&sr=1-5

7-Ein Lied von Rahman geschrieben: Aden (German Edition) (German) Paperback – April 28, 2015 at this link: http://www.amazon.com/Ein-Lied-von-Rahman-geschrieben/dp/1511930101/ref=sr_1_6?s=books&ie=UTF8&qid=1441596254&sr=1-6&pebp=1441596262908&perid=0JEQRACTBPJGCEQYJYMC

8- Medecin de chefs: Une collection de veritables histoires (French Edition) (French)Paperback – June 8, 2015 at this link:
http://www.amazon.com/Medecin-chefs-collection-veritables-histoires/dp/1514269430/ref=sr_1_2?s=books&ie=UTF8&qid=1441596378&sr=1-2

9- Greats on the top: "Secrets of success and financial intelligence and access to billions" (1) (Arabic Edition) (Arabic) Paperback – July 27, 2015 at this link: http://www.amazon.com/Greats-top-financial-intelligence-billions/dp/1515248062/ref=sr_1_1?s=books&ie=UTF8&qid=1441596658&sr=1-1

www.ingramcontent.com/pod-product-compliance
Lightning Source LLC
Chambersburg PA
CBHW041101180526
45172CB00001B/54